RAWLLY SIMPLE

~

A Guide To Eating What We Are Designed To Eat

C.B. Thompson

© Love & Light Publishing 2018

All rights reserved. No part of this book may be reproduced in any nature with-out written permission from the publisher, except in the case of quoted material identified within the book.

Love & Light Publishing
www.loveandlightpublishing.com

Author: C.B. Thompson
ISBN: 9781983133190
Imprint: Independently published

First, I would like to thank Dr. Robert Morse ND for generously sharing his knowledge through his books and freely on YouTube. Dr. Morse is fundamentally the reason for this book, and for turning my life around. I am eternally grateful for your profound knowledge and wisdom.

I also thank those who lovingly guided me to find Dr. Morse in my darkest times. You will always be remembered in my heart and soul.

Table of Contents

Introduction

This is your wake-up call.

I won't tell you it is easy.

I will tell you it will be the best decision you ever make.

I have no problem going out on a limb and stating that if you implement this diet and lifestyle to the fullest extent, you will have never felt so good in your life, never. Not even when you were born.
I will say it again though, it won't be easy. We have all been brainwashed for as long as you have been alive and your parents before that, and their parents and so on down the line.

At some point it was likely a necessity of survival. This will be true if you live in the northern hemisphere. It is no longer an excuse though, as we have access to pretty well everything we could ever possibly need to survive, delivered all over the world, right to your friendly neighborhood grocery store.

So, this cold weather survival excuse is no longer valid, hasn't been for at least 50 years, and likely longer.

There is no need to eat meat or dairy or grains/breads and pasta to survive in the winter. There is no need to can food to last the winter. Those days are gone, thankfully.

Unfortunately, so many people have forgotten about the fresh produce section of the grocery store. I find that it is usually right at the entrance to the store and most people walk right past it, heading to the processed food sections of the store. Guess what makes up 80% (at least) of the grocery store foot print... processed food... that's really sad.

Meat and fresh produce make up the other 20% or less of the stores floor plan.

I have no problem with frozen fruits and vegetables, their very handy for storing food in your house so you're not having to run out to the store every 2 or 3 days.

Unfortunately, the large majority of the grocery store chains have 80% or more of their dedicated floor space allocated for processed food.

Now, if you haven't guessed it by now, this book is about raw food living, hence the title; *Rawlly Simple*.

I have converted myself from a staunch meat and potatoes eating machine, and a lot of junk food, into a raw food loving machine.

The difference in the way you feel is unbelievable, and in the following pages of the book, you will start to see what I mean.

Join me if you will...

In Love & Light,
C.B. Thompson

Chapter 1

Let me begin with eliminating the myths around diets.

Anyone heard this one?

We **need** to eat protein.

That statement alone is likely the biggest cause of most of the issues with human health on the planet.

We don't *need* to eat protein. We *choose* to eat protein. I'm talking about every kind of protein, including nuts.

I just heard a whole bunch of "ya, but..."

But what?

What about Vitamin B12 deficiencies? How do I get iron? Won't I lose all my muscle mass? Doesn't protein give me energy? Won't my blood sugar be out of whack if I don't eat protein?

I'm sure there are more but I'm also sure you get the point.

Here is the big misunderstanding about consuming protein, be it from meat, nuts, Greek yogurt and so on. The body cannot utilize protein straight from the source as you eat it, it has to break the protein structure down into the basic elements that were used to create the protein structure in the first place. Meaning, your body has to use a lot of digestive process to break down the food you ate as a protein structure back into the Amino Acids that were used in the first place to create the protein structure.

So, you see, it is Amino Acids that you want to consume to provide your body with the proper elements to create protein structures within the body.

Just Google it if you don't believe me. Search online and let me know if I am lying. Do a little research and see what Amino Acids are for, or, what happens to protein with your body digests and breaks it down.

Are you also starting to see that protein isn't used for energy? Protein is a structure of the body. Sugar is energy, preferably fructose or glucose.

Now, again I hear a "ya, but..."

What about animals that eat meat? Don't they get their nutrition and energy from eating meat?

Do you fancy yourself to be a carnivore? Not likely.

Also, next time your watching some nature show and a carnivore catches its meal, watch closely what part of the catch they eat first, and prefer to eat. I'll give you a hint, it won't be the muscle...

I bet though, that you consider yourself to be an omnivore. Well, you would be among the majority of those on the planet who think that as well. Now, pause for thought for just a moment. If that were the case, that we are omnivores, and we have thought this for thousands of years, then why are we not getting healthier and living longer?

Let me ask you this question, do we look like omnivores?

Do you look like a bear? Do you look like a pig? Do you look like a dog? Maybe a chicken?

Truthfully the omnivores eat more plant-based food than protein. Most of them only eat other animals when they want some fat.

What species do we most resemble inside and what is their main diet? Take your time in researching their diet on the internet, I'll be right here when you get back.

Notice how I stated to search "their" diet on the internet?

That's because I'm pretty certain that you are going to choose gorilla's, orangutans or chimpanzees as the species that we are most similar to.

Now, what is their primary diet? Whether or not you darted off to the computer to get the answer I'll tell you, it's fruit.

The main source of food for the species that resembles us internally and a little on the outside the most like humans is fruit.

Just think of the size of a full grown male silverback gorilla and how powerful it is, and what is its main source of food, that it would choose above and beyond all other choices of food?

Fruit.

So, does a hulking gorilla need protein to survive?

Nope.

Does a mighty elephant need protein to become huge and powerful?

Nope.

Now, I would like to clarify one thing again. Even omnivores eat very little protein, their diets will consist mostly of plant-based food. Protein is without a doubt very hard on the body to digest.

So, I don't want to belabour the point, but you can see that protein is not a good source of food for humans. We already know that the medical industry states that protein is tough on our poor old kidneys. I will get into that in more detail later.

If anything, you decided to seriously look at protein and consider eliminating or significantly reduce your consumption of protein in your diet, and never read another page in this book, then I would be forever grateful and my work here is done. Your body would also be very grateful, as the assault on it would be partially over, at least the most damaging one for your kidneys.

So, for those who believe that we need protein in our diets to survive, think Amino Acids. These are the true building blocks of our bodies.

So, I'm sure you are just asking the question, "where can we get Amino Acids?" I'm glad you asked, why fruit and veggies of course!

Fruits and veggies are packed with Amino Acids, how else do primates and herbivores get so huge and powerful?

Now, after that exhausting rant, what's next?

Dairy.

Oh ya, I said it, dairy.

What ever made us think that we needed to consume milk from anything but our mother as a baby? And, why do we need to keep consuming it after we have been weaned off of it? Does any other species on Earth continue to consume their mothers milk after they should be weaned?

Hopefully I didn't hear anyone say yes.

Of course not, what makes us think that we need to keep consuming milk products?

Oh ya, that's right, this crazy belief that we need tons of calcium and the best source is cow's milk... not even remotely close to our species... and on top of that we boil the heck out of it and turn it almost into plastic. Then we consider it an extremely healthy source of food...

Are you starting to see the insanity here?

Are you starting to see the crazy way that we have created this narrative that no other species on Earth follows?

All other species on Earth eats exactly what is natural to them.

On top of that, what other specie cooks their food before eating it? That's correct! No other specie cooks their food before eating it, they don't have to, it's exactly as it needs to be to provide them with the proper nutrition and energy... more importantly, the energy!

So, we humans have gone off the deep end with our food, and don't we love our food!

Let's recap shall we, before we go on?

We eat something that our bodies cannot use in the form that it's eaten, and more times than not, we cook the heck out of it until there is no energy left in it to take. Then we wash it down with something that baby cows consume to grow before being weaned off to eat grass... is something here not sitting right with you?

Oh ya, by the way, cooking... what do you think happens to the chemistry of the food when it's cooked? Do you think that it is the same as it was before it was cooked? I won't keep you in suspense, it's not. It has been changed, and whatever nutrition is stated on the label is before it was cooked... oh

ya, that's what you just read, the nutritional label is
pre-cooked nutrition... the misinformation gets
deeper and deeper...

To be clear, I was just as duped as you, but
thankfully I had significant health issues which
shook me to my knees and made me seek the truth
about what I was doing to myself.

So, I don't want everyone to think that I am casting
blame on the farmers, doctors and the nutritionists
for all this trouble, I am not. They are just as in the
dark as you and I were before realizing the truth.

The problem I have is with the people higher up the
totem pole that know the truth and keep pushing
this agenda of telling us that protein, dairy, grains,
and so on are critical to our health. The famous food
guide if you will.

Oh, they are critical to our health all right...

People at the top of the pyramid know that this is
not good for us, but because they profit from selling
the food, the medical care we need and the
pharmaceuticals that we need to take to ease the
symptoms that consuming incorrect food gives us,
makes them all mighty rich. So why would you start
to tell the truth?

There's not a lot of money to be made in the truth.

What's the truth you ask? Well, I will get into that
later, but here's a teaser. No illness, no need to visit
the dentist, no need for pills. This won't happen
overnight, but if you commit to the diet meant for

humans, then it is possible, and you will feel like you have never felt before, and I mean that, like you have **never** felt before. More on that later.

Ok, before jumping into the next chapter I will briefly touch on the other bad choices.

Grains.

Ya, it's true, you don't need it. It really doesn't do anything for you. What nutrition and energy comes from grains?

Do you really think you need to eat your oatmeal in the morning to help you get started with your day? Sticks to your ribs, right? Ya, right, exactly what it does, sticks. It's like eating glue that gets stuck and slows down in digesting so it begins to ferment/rot and gets impacted in your body.

That just reminded me about something very important that I will detail more later, but something that I want to say here as well to emphasize for all those that still think they need to eat meat. Since I have already mentioned how difficult it is for your body to digest meat, this really slows down digestion and this is why you feel fuller longer after eating meat. Well, there is a significant side effect to having slow digestion of meat. It's essentially rotting inside your body... it's called putrefaction and it is as nasty as it sounds... wonder now why people have problems with bacteria and parasites???

Sorry for that side step, but it's a very important detail that few people realize.

So, grains, what are they good for! Absolutely nothing!

Yes, I totally agree, they taste so darn good as breads and pasta, but you are really not doing yourself any good consuming them.

Again, they slow down digestion and ferment/rot, bringing the fungus family into action to deal with the fermentation.

Are you itchy, rashing and a little on the smelly side? How are your feet? Good and stinky and maybe a little bit of athletes' foot?

How about some warts?

That would be our fungus family paying you a visit because you invited them over for dinner. More on that later.

I really have said more than enough about the myths of nutrition and health.

I didn't touch the super-food myth, you know what I mean, kale and such. We'll get more into that later.

I think that is good enough for now for you to mull over. These have been the biggest ones that have hurt humans more than anything else and if you simply eliminated all of the things I talked about above and became a raw food vegan then you will have created a life for yourself that will change you in ways that you can't imagine!

Why stop there when there is a whole other level to health and vitality?

Join me in the coming chapters and learn what true health is all about!

Chapter 2

I want to get back to asking the question, "Are we crazy?!?"

I alluded to this a little bit in the previous chapter and I will expand upon it further here.

What makes our Standard American Diet (SAD) so crazy?

Does anyone else see the irony that the acronym for the typical diet is SAD???

Anyway, the crazy part goes back to what I wrote about cooking our food before we eat it and eating all the food that is not meant for us to eat.

So, think really hard about what animal or anything at all that cooks their food before they eat it.

For those that are having a hard time to think of us humans as in the same class as animals, get over yourself. Once you have finished reading this book you will hopefully think differently about the way we eat and treat others.

Ok, that should be enough time to think... because the answer is simple, no other animal or anything on planet earth, other than humans, cooks their food before eating it.

Nothing.

We are the absolute craziest things on this planet.

And we are supposed to be the highest intelligence...

Here is something that will be new to most but is really critical.

We should not really think about our food with worrying about nutrition first and whether or not we are getting all the vitamins and minerals needed to live.

Most other living things have a mono diet, meaning that they typically eat one type of food. Now I am not aware of any food on the planet that has every type of vitamin and mineral in it that would be complete.

So, what is that really telling us.

That nutrition is not everything.

Well then, what is?

Energy.

Energy is everywhere and everything and without that, we would be dead.

So, yes, we get energy from our food and from everything around us, but for now this book will focus on the energy that we get from food.

So, if horses, gorillas and elephants can eat basically one source of food and be that healthy, then I would think that we can have fewer food choices and live quite nicely as well.

Can you just imagine what a grocery store would look like if all we did was eat what we are designed to eat?

I look very forward to that happy day.

So, what is the primary source of energy for humans?

Sugar.

Yup, the very thing that almost every doctor and nutrition guru has told us is bad for us.

Why do they do this? I really don't know but as you likely read earlier, I have my suspicion that I know where the source comes from.

For those of you who are ready to stick me with an "I told you so" knife, yes, I mean sugar is the energy source of humans. Do you think I mean white processed sugar in a can of soda? Of course, I don't mean any old kind of sugar, that would be crazy. Yes, that kind of sugar will give you some energy, but it will be short lived and you will crash hard when your body uses whatever it can from it. No, I am meaning fructose and/or glucose as the preferred sugar and fructose as the best sugar.

Ok, lets dive a little deeper into the cooked food versus uncooked food train of thought.

What do you think the level of energy would be from a cooked vegetable versus a raw vegetable? This could be a pot of boiled carrots that are now nice and mushy for eating. I'm not going to get technical in this book, and you can look up energy from food on the internet. Not calories, real, natural energy. All I will tell you is that cooked food will have significantly less energy than raw food, not to mention that you have changed the chemistry of the food from cooking it.

So, to me, I am interested in getting energy from the food I eat. This means I need to eat food that contains sugar, simple sugar, and food high in natural energy.

This is something that is likely quite new to people, that there is natural energy to food, and when you cook food, the natural energy of the food is reduced.

Just think about it for a minute, was the food not alive before you cooked it?

Also, as stated earlier, sugar is the required source of energy for humans.

It's not just any old kind of sugar either for us humans, it's simple sugar that our bodies want. The only natural simple sugars that exist are fructose (from fruit), glucose (think veggies) and lactose (milk).

All other sugars are considered complex sugars and are more difficult for our bodies to digest and can lead to health issues such as diabetes and obesity.

Now, in my opinion, the best sugar for a human is fructose, as study and experience from Dr. Morse (ND) has shown that fructose does not need insulin as a carrier into the cell. Glucose needs insulin to cross into the cell.

This has been proven at Dr. Morse's clinic from diabetics who do not need to use insulin when they eat strictly fruit, but when they eat vegetables, they then need to use insulin.

There may be some glucose loading at first when they just eat fructose, but over time and under control, they will get to the point where they can eat only fruit and need no insulin. It's true.

This clearly demonstrates that glucose is an inferior sugar to fructose for humans.

Up until now you have likely been very sceptical about my statements. I accept that.

So, lets get even more real for you.

Let's stop talking technical and strip it right down, right now, right here.

How do you think a really good way would be to tell what type of food it is that your body really wants?

It's simple really.

Think about any kind of food that is your favorite and tell me if you could; 1. Eat it raw, and 2. Eat it plain.

Yup, I just went there!

If you think that steak is your favorite food, can you eat it raw and could you eat it plain?

Ok, let's make this simpler, because I just heard someone scoff at that, saying that eating raw meat is disgusting.

Ok, fair enough, go ahead and cook your steak to your desired level, mine used to be medium rare just in case you were interested...

So, it's cooked to perfection, I hope you didn't add any spices, marinade or sauce... that wasn't part of the deal, you have to eat it plain. Do you really love that steak now? Or, was it the fact that it was cooked and covered or flavoured with something to the point that you didn't really taste the meat anyway?

Now, ask yourself the same question with a bowl of pineapple, or mango, or a banana?

Do you need to cook the fruit or add anything to it to make it taste better?

I didn't think you did. Ya sure, you could sprinkle stuff on it if you wanted to, but truthfully, you could eat an apple or banana just as it is, couldn't you, and of course, the majority of people do just that.

Now, lets go deeper...

Veggies.

Be totally honest with yourself here.

How many of you can eat veggies without making a salad and putting dressing and other additives on it?

Can you eat a salad plain?

Hopefully you are starting to see the point I am trying to make.

That is, that we mask the food that we have been eating because we don't actually like the taste of the food.

This should be a huge wake up call for many.

I actually ask you to put down this book and really think about it. Think about what we have been doing for all these years, that we have been taught, that we do without thinking.

We mask the food so that we will eat it, the very food that is not healthy for us and that we would never eat if it wasn't cooked or smothered in flavors to the point that we will eat it.

So, this goes hand in hand with a point I made earlier about thinking that we need protein.

We *choose* to eat the food we are not designed to eat, and we fool ourselves into eating the food we are not designed to eat by cooking it or masking it with things that make us eat it.

So, I think that is enough for this chapter, now we will explore what is going on in your body when you eat the wrong foods.

Chapter 3

Now that we have discussed the points of what food is best for the human design and why, it's time to state what happens to the body when the wrong food is consumed.

I need to preface this chapter with a quick chemistry lesson.

When it comes to the human body, there are only two sides of chemistry that we are concerned with. Acids and Base.

Acids break down humans and base builds, in very simple terms.

Yes, being too Alkaline is a bad thing, but 99.9% of the health issues humans have are created from the acid side of chemistry. Ok, I grabbed the 99.9% out of the air, but I am not aware of anyone suffering from being over Alkaline.

The point I am making is that the majority of known major causes of death come from eating the wrong foods and creating the wrong chemistry in the human body.

What makes it worse, is that the medical industry uses mainly acidic medical means to treat their defined dis-eases.

The worst offender that I can think of is chemo... this is like using battery acid to fix something. How do you think it will turn out?

Getting back to what happens in our bodies, when we eat food that is not meant for humans, our bodies are programmed to process it. There is no off switch or bypass valve if you suddenly realize that you should not have eaten something. Your body will process it.

Now, the body uses chemical processes to digest food, this is not something new and most of you will know this. What you may not know is that the seemingly simple act of digesting food creates acid by-products in the body that need to be eliminated.

So, if the food you are consuming is difficult for your body to break down and utilize, then that means that more of these acid chemical processes are needed to be created and more needs to be removed.

Here's another fun fact... we are already born into this world with less than 100% functioning bodies, so when the wrong food is eaten, we are not helping our bodies at all.

Why can I say that our bodies are not 100% perfect when we are born? Well, take a look at your parents before you were born. Are they 100% healthy? No? Well then, that would explain your predicament.

It is not a stretch at all to state that everyone has compromised kidneys or bowels to some degree, which affects their ability to eliminate the acidic wastes from their bodies to ensure that you are a lean running machine.

Here is another critical fact that most people will not be aware of. What is the main function of the kidneys? I'll cut right to the chase. To filter and eliminate cellular or metabolic waste from the body.

Now, here is another critical part, most people believe that the kidneys only filter the blood...

There is a system in our bodies that few know anything about, it's called the Lymphatic System. It has many functions, but I would argue that it's most important function is to carry cellular or metabolic waste from the body and eliminate it either through the kidneys, or the skin. Obviously eliminating waste through the kidneys and ultimately in the Urine is the preferred route, but if the kidneys are not functioning properly then the body has to do what it has to do and the skin is known as the third kidney for a reason.

So, with all this in mind, let's get back to what happens in our bodies when we eat the wrong foods, and when our bodies cannot properly dispose of the waste products.

Well, we know that if we are not functioning properly we start to not feel well and then end up at the doctors where they tell us we have some type of dis-ease. The main reason they do this is because, unfortunately, the majority of doctors don't know what is truly wrong. They use your symptoms to draw a conclusion from the knowledge they learned in school, or from learning and researching the dis-ease from peers or databases.

The scary part here is that the vast majority of "diseases" they have created has nothing to do with what causes the symptoms, so they have little chance of curing the so-called "disease". All they can hope to do is treat the symptoms to make you feel better, but as you can hopefully realize right now, you are not curing the cause of the symptoms.

What's even worse, is the means of treating the symptoms.

Pharmaceuticals.

So, not only are you not going to get your remedy, you are going to get prescribed some treatment that will more than likely suppress the symptoms, causing the part of your body that was giving you symptoms to be even more compromised... but you won't even be aware of it. That is until the part of your body that is having the trouble can't be suppressed any longer and then look out!

The disease, or symptoms, will seem to come back even worse... wonder why???

Likely your doctor will tell you that your body is becoming immune to the drug and that you need to change the type of drug you're on or be prescribed a higher dosage.

Does this sound familiar at all???

Ok, one quick thing as I got off the tracks a little, but this information I just shared is very important background to know going forward. I want to be very clear, I am not bashing doctors here, they just have not been trained properly, so if there is anyone to blame, it would be the organization that trains doctors, and likely even higher above that, because they have to be, or had to have known that this insanity is not working... however, do they know it does not work??? I'll leave that for you to decide. All I will say is that the medical industry is a major money maker, and I will leave it at that.

Ok, back to what happens in your body when you can't eliminate waste properly.

Remember back to the two sides of chemistry and remember what type of chemistry is waste products and by-products in the body, specifically cellular or metabolic waste? Right, acidic chemistry. So, if this waste is acidic and your body is not able to properly eliminate it out, what do you think acids do. Well, acids are corrosive right? Right, and if these wastes are not being eliminated, what might these corrosive acids be doing to the cells that make up everything in your body. Right again! The acidic wastes are breaking down your cells, or what may be called cancer.

So, to quickly link the previous discussion on treating symptoms. What do you think the majority of prescribed drugs do in treating symptoms, suppress the symptoms right? Do you believe that they eliminate the cause of the symptoms through the designed parts of your body that dispose of these acidic wastes that are causing the pain and discomfort that show up as symptoms?

Nope.

They "make the pain go away", well, not out of your body they don't!

These drugs make the pain and discomfort of the symptoms go away, but the actual problem (acids) don't go anywhere and now you think they are gone and go back to your normal life… if you can.

So, you can see how it is all related, and by not addressing the cause of the symptoms and only treating the symptoms, it makes it worse by keeping the acids in your body longer, causing more damage and potentially leading to cancer, or, if cancer is already present, makes it worse and seemingly spreading.

Now, cancer is a pretty serious topic to be talking about being a result of not eliminating acidic waste, however, it is true. Let's discuss another popular ailment or symptom of humans, arthritis. Can you guess what causes it? Auto-immune diseases, right?

Nope.

Another indication that the doctors don't understand what causes these so called dis-eases. The problem is inflammation and degradation, which could only come from an acidic environment, I would think. Now where did these acids come from??? You get the point, right?

Now, I can't list out every symptom that you would experience from your body not eliminating waste, but you should be able to start to get a picture of what it means to eat the wrong foods when your body is not functioning properly.

Quick reminder, in order to break down the food
you eat, your body uses chemical processes that
need to be eliminated and not all of these wastes go
into the toilet when you do the #2, if you know what
I mean. There is also a lot of cellular activity taking
place to break down and digest the food, which
creates acidic waste that must be eliminated through
the kidney's (preferably) or out through the skin
(not preferred).

The bottom line is that if you're not eliminating the
acidic wastes out of your body properly, you are at
great risk of these acids breaking down the cells and
becoming what doctors refer to as cancer, which is
just the destruction of a normal cell.

Also, as we stated earlier, these acidic wastes aren't
just the potential cause of cancer, think of any disease and then think about what is causing the pain
and discomfort, or the dis-ease of the body.

The bottom line, again, is that acids are corrosive,
and if left in the body long enough, and
concentrated enough, they will break down cells in
the body. Remember that everything in your body is
made up of cells and two fluids - blood and lymph.

So, enough said, onto the next chapter.

Chapter 4

I would like to continue on in further detail, and discussion, about the cellular or metabolic wastes generated in your body.

The importance of this cannot be understated as to what it is doing to the health of this planet. This, of course, is when the kidneys are not functioning properly.

Yes, the colon plays an important part in your health, and it needs to be healthy as well, but if you focus on getting your kidneys healthy, the rest will work out fine.

Now, lets dive deeper into cellular or metabolic waste, where it comes from and how it is made.

As mentioned earlier, your body uses chemical processes to break down food when you digest it. Most of that waste goes through the digestive tract and out through what we know as the #2 route. That is referred to as digestive waste.

Now, some of that food, or nutrients, ends up in the blood and in your cells as food for the cells to function. I hope you can agree that every cell in your body, be it a skin cell, muscle cell or a bone cell needs food to survive.

Now, what if the food they are getting is not ideal for their function? Well, they wouldn't function properly, or they wouldn't use the food completely and would need to eliminate the waste.

Where does the waste go?

This is a question most will get wrong, unfortunately, and they cannot be blamed. I would have easily gotten it wrong not so long ago.

For those who have been paying attention as they have been reading will likely be getting the sense of what the answer is.

It's the blood of course!

Wrong!

Yes, most people would have said that the waste products go into the blood and then the blood is cleaned through the kidneys and all is good... no, that would be bad... if the blood becomes acidic to a certain degree, you will be in big trouble. The blood needs to remain alkaline for you to survive.

If you have acidic blood, think minutes of survival. Minutes.

I want to add an important point, cells in your body will make waste regardless if they get food from the blood or not. Think about walking or exercising, or just plain cell multiplication. When cells do any of the things I just mentioned, they are using energy and creating waste.
All you are made up of is cells… your alive right? Why wouldn't your cells be alive, need food – energy – and have the need to eliminate waste?
Of course your cells are alive, need food and need to eliminate waste… but here is the real problem…

do you think that the cells in your body can excuse themselves for a minute, travel somewhere in your body, and find a bathroom to use…?
That's pretty obvious, the cells in you body don't go anywhere to go to the bathroom, that is the job of the massive Lymph System.

Food = Blood / Kitchen; Waste handling = Lymph System / Bathroom.

The waste products go into the Lymphatic system, always have, always will... unless... your Lymphatic system is compromised and then you're in trouble. The majority of cancers happen in the Lymph system, look it up or ask your doctor.

So, when a cell in your body eats and poops, yes, even your cells do the same thing as you, the poop does not go back into the food source... do you poop in your fridge or your kitchen? I didn't think so, you go to the bathroom in the... bathroom! The sewer system!

So, your house and your body are very similar. You have a kitchen for food and a sewer for waste. You body have blood for food and a Lymph system (or sewer system) for waste.

No one poops in their kitchen and your body does not poop in its blood.

Now, to repeat, your cells also create waste when they are just being normal, being active and doing their thing. This might be hard for people to visualize so let's make it more real. If you exercise in the gym or go for a jog, would you say your cells are working? I hope you would. And since they are working, they are using energy, right? Right. Now, if they are using energy (eating) they must be producing waste? Yes, they are, and those wastes will be acidic and must be removed from the cell or those wastes will break down the cell because they are acidic.

A favorite analogy of mine is to consider what happens if you don't change a baby's diaper in a timely fashion. What happens to the baby's skin and what does the baby do? All new parents are well aware of what I am saying. The baby cries and the lower end of the baby is red and rashing.

So, what is happening here?

What is happening is that the waste products (pee and/or poop) is acidic and is breaking down the skin cells because the pee and/or poop is in contact with the skin cells and acids burn and destroy.

The exact same thing is happening at the cellular level with the waste products of the cells activity. If the waste products are not removed in a timely fashion... they break down the cell and you get what the doctors call cancer, which can come with pain, just like the baby's bottom.

This all makes sense, right?

I'm not saying anything totally crazy, right? Well, it is crazy when you think that doctors don't seem to be able to connect the dots and figure this out.

It's just simple chemistry and physics.

Waste is acidic, if it cannot be eliminated from the body through the kidneys or the skin it is burning up what ever it is in contact with, and that burning of the cells is called cancer.

So, this does not happen as fast as you might be thinking because the body has more than one line of defence... it's almost as though the body was designed knowing it was going to get abused... I don't know about you but that seems sad...

The body can deploy various means of chemical processes to attempt to neutralize the acidity of the waste. There is cholesterol, there are steroids, and there is calcium (think ant-acids). Plus, there is good old water. So, the body does its best to keep the acids neutral if it can't be eliminated, but over time, these processes can't combat all the built-up waste and eventually the cells are going to break down because the waste is getting backed up into the cell itself and then you have cancer.

Even if the cell gets the waste out but it has only gone as far as just outside the cellular wall, that acidic waste can break down the cell wall and again we have cancer.

This can get fairly complex and drawn out and I don't want to bore you with the details, however, this is critical for you to understand because you are not going to get this information from your doctor.

The bottom line is that your body creates waste at all levels and functions and if those wastes are not eliminated through the kidneys or the skin, your going to find that you are having health issues.

Just something to think about.

Do you have rashes on your skin? Do you have skin issues? What might that be? Well, just under or on the surface of your skin are acidic wastes that your skin is not eliminating properly. This could be because you don't sweat easily, because you have low thyroid function.

Here is another one to think about, your joints are sore or you have been diagnosed with arthritis. Why would this be? Can you come up with your own answer with all that you have read? Would it be because there are acidic wastes trapped in and around your joints breaking down the tissues? Is your body producing a natural immune response to try and neutralize the acids and causing pain and swelling because the wastes cannot be moved out and eliminated?

See what is happening here?

Your body is not attacking itself with some crazy made up auto-immune disease!

The body is protecting itself and there is only so much it can do when we are consuming the wrong foods and then we have compromised kidneys and skin so we are not eliminating properly.

This is the sad state of affairs and is what is happening to people today.

We all need to give our poor bodies a break and stop this insanity of eating proteins, dairy, grains and anything other that fruit and some vegetables.

What you will find is that as you eat these foods, raw, your body will get the food it wants, and it will be able to spend more time fixing itself.

Herbs need to be considered, but at this time we won't get into it and perhaps not at all in this book, but just know that herbs are an important part of the healing method and there is much to learn.

Please get a mental picture in your mind that there is this sewer system in your body that, if everything was normal, would be carrying away the acidic wastes from your cells and in between the cells through a very large network of vessels and nodes (that further break down the acids into less acidic waste - more towards the alkaline side), which all lead to the kidneys, which process this waste and transfers it into the bladder and out through the urine.

That is the simple version of what happens and is good enough to know what is happening and you will already be farther ahead of your doctor in knowing how the body eliminates metabolic / cellular waste from the body.

The other amazing thing to remember is that it is the body that does the healing, not the food. A cut on your finger heals right? Right, and the same thing happens inside you and with your cells. The body will heal itself. If you're pretty acidic, it will take longer, if your lymph system, kidneys and skin are compromised, it will take longer.

I hope that this is getting through to you.

The things that doctors prescribe to you do not heal you, your body does.

Chemo does not heal you, no way in the world does chemo heal you... it is an acid, and what do we already know that acids do?

You already know, if not, go back through this book.

So, if the doctor wants to prescribe a radiation and chemo treatment, run out the door and never look back.

If you went immediately to a raw food diet of fruits, berries or melons, your body would do the rest. Now, I must point out that I cannot provide medical advice, so please seek the advice of a qualified natural medicine practitioner who does not prescribe supplements, or a protein diet. Take the time to find a doctor that will provide you with common sense care that goes along with what you have learned in this book.

I am here to merely provide you with information to educate you and hopefully make you see the world from a new perspective and makes sense.

The body heals itself, and if we get out of the way and stop harming it with the wrong foods and environment, it will fix itself. Even the medical industry can't argue that the body doesn't heal itself and it's the pharmaceutical that do it...

Drugs only treat symptoms, we already went over that.

I could go on and on describing every made up, so-called disease known to man, but I won't. Why? Because the cause for all of these issues is the same, the same cause and effect.
It is all caused from acids in the body, and a comprised elimination system.
Period, that simple. Get that in your head and you are done, you can stop reading this book, head out to the local market and pick up some fresh and organic fruits and vegetables and start snacking!

In all seriousness though, this is the truth as far as I can explain it to you.
I can completely understand that it is difficult to trust me, everywhere you turn, some ad, some video or professional is telling you that you have to eat protein or dairy or whatever to survive and the reason you are not feeling well, or tired or whatever is because you are just missing some vital and critical mineral or something... all I can do is tell you from my own personal experience, and from many who all tell you about it on YouTube or on their blogs, is that it is all untrue.

Give your body a break and just try a raw diet for a week and see how you feel.

Chapter 5

I could go on and on about dis-eases and what is going on, but I won't.

I know I spent a long time on cancer, but the causes of all issues in the body – even neurological issues – are all the same and the remedy is all the same, so I don't need to go on and on for chapter after chapter saying the same things in the end.
I will say that Dr. Morse recommends the berry family of fruits for healing neurological issues.
So, if you have MS, or ALS or anything where the neurons aren't firing like they should be, start eating the berries and think about looking into some herbs for the brain and nerve system.
For that, please consult the professionals, I don't want to turn this into a book on protocol's.

I also don't want this to be a long book, there is no reason for it.
I have told you about what the wrong foods do to your body, now it is your turn to see why I am telling you this.

Go out to the store right after you have finished reading this chapter and go get yourself some fresh and organic (if you can) fruit and vegetables.

Get whatever fruits and veggies you like, you want to go into this with a positive attitude, and one that will work.
Please try and go one week eating only raw fruit and see how you feel. After the week you can eat

your normal diet if you want to see how you feel from that.

Use a journal to write how you feel everyday, at the end of the week on fruit, and then write how you feel on your regular diet.
It's important to do that so you can see the difference.

Do you get heartburn easily? Do you get congested?

See how you feel for a week eating only raw compared to your regular diet.
Then, try it again, maybe this time just eat vegetables.
Experiment, it's important, and always write down how you feel.

Do you have a sore shoulder or wrist?
Eat only raw fruit for a week or two, then see how your shoulder or wrist feels. Just as sore? A little less? Can you get full motion out of it?

How about your knees?

See what I am getting at? Just try it, it's only a week, what do you have to lose?

Now, I am fully sensitive to people's schedules or needs or family pressures, so pick a time when it is most convenient and then give it a go. Don't put it off until your New Year's Resolution if you're reading this in the month of February… if you are really serious about changing your life and healing your body, then figure it out and give it a go for one week.

You won't regret it.

Ok, what I want to do here before I wrap up this book is just mention what fruits are more powerful that others for healing.

Grapes and lemons are two of the best for cleaning out your body.

Let me be clear about something, what I am writing about in this book is that you are going to do a detox, but a proper one. No pills, no shakes or bars, just raw fruit and some veggies.

You can juice them, blender them up in smoothies or just pick them up and eat them, but please eat them raw.
And also, do not mix fruits with vegetables.
This is simply because of digestive speeds. You will digest fruits faster that most, if not all other foods.
And also, do not mix melons with other food, even fruit. Melons digest so fast that if you eat a big summertime meal of meat, corn and potatoes, and then finish it off with watermelon, that watermelon will start to ferment in your body because you body can digest it so much faster than the other food all mixed up in your belly.
However, most people might not even realize, because they have likely washed down the main course with a beer! Or two…

Some of the gentler fruits are banana's, mango's, peaches, pears and so on, what would be considered the less acidic fruits… which just brought me to a very important thought, and a good one to end this

book on so that you have all the knowledge you will
ever need to navigate through healing yourself,
well, there are two more items, and here they are:
The issue with your body getting acidic is not from
eating acid foods, or at least not how the foods start
off in your body when you consume them, it is how
the food digests!
All of the foods that I stated earlier in the book that
are bad for you digest as acidic waste, that is the
important part to remember here! The waste, or ash,
from consuming meats, dairy, grains, eggs and so
on is acidic. Fruits and vegetables do not leave
acidic waste, or ash, after digestion, that is why
fruits and vegetables can heal you, the waste
product of fruits and vegetables is alkaline.

I am glad to have gotten that into this book, it is the
whole point of this discussion.

There is acid ash food and there is alkaline ash
food. Or another way of putting it is that when your
body does its chemical digestion process, the end
result is an acidic waste left behind, or an alkaline
waste.
You choose which waste you would like to
process…

Here is the second important thing I want to end this
book on – healing crisis.
This will be absolutely new to many, if not all of
you.
When you really get into a raw food diet, you may
start to feel symptoms that will make you believe
you are getting sick from the raw diet, or that your
symptoms are getting worse.
Now, this is a critical item.

The raw diet, and your bodies ability to heal itself,
may make you feel even more uncomfortable at
times, and, it may even be right away.
Please do not panic.
Unless you feel like you are in too much pain to
continue, try to push through it. Once you get
through the pain and discomfort, you are done.

What is likely happening here is that the fruits and
your bodies natural ability to heal itself is stirring
up the acidic wastes and causing pain, inflammation
and general, or specific, symptoms, that you will
decipher as some disease, or that you can't eat fruit.

Please, this is the time to put the knowledge from
this book into practice and really ask yourself if
fruit or vegetables could cause a disease?

I would hope that after all that I have explained that
you would know the answer is that it is not possible
for a natural food to cause a disease, because,
diseases are made up, and simply describe a
symptom or effect of some inflammation or
degradation in the body.

Fruit or vegetables cannot cause any so-called
diseases, only acids can.

Now, if you are in serious or life-threatening pain or
discomfort, then please seek medical help. You may
be more acidic or in worse shape than you
originally thought, and the raw diet and the bodies
natural healing ability has been too strong.

Once things have settled down, then take it a bit
slower, know your limits and play within it!

But don't worry, you can do this, and your body
will do its best to heal.
You may need some herbs or pharmaceutical pain
medication for a bit to help you get through the
early part, but do you best to go only fruit or
vegetable at first and see how your body reacts.

For those of you, like people with diabetes for
example, will likely need the help of a good and
understanding doctor to help control their bodies
reaction to a new diet, and to help wean them off of
the medication as they go.

But don't be afraid, you can do this, there is nothing
to be afraid of.
If you want to be afraid of anything, be afraid of
putting your life in the hands of a medical doctor
who has no idea about healing… only treating you
through a possibly painful and untimely death.

Sorry to be so stark about that comment, but it is
true, I watched my own father pass away from
cancer at the hands of doctors that, unfortunately,
had no clue and although were very caring people,
prescribed treatments to him that lead to his death.

So, I am fully aware of the results of a poor diet and
a medical system that cannot cure.

So, if you want to be aggressive about this journey,
then go on a 10-day grape diet and see what
happens.
I have a feeling a lot will happen, some good, some
not so fun. But hopefully you will feel much better
as a result of it.

If you want to slow it down a bit, then go with the less aggressive fruits or eat fruit for breakfast, a salad at lunch and then either fruit again for supper, or another veggie meal.

Play around with it and have some fun with it, that is what it is all about anyway!

So, I will end it off here, my intention wasn't to be the encyclopedia of healing. I just wanted to get your attention, tell you, in plain language, the truth about the typical diet, and how you can find your remedy.

This book is just meant to be a launching pad into your new lifelong journey into a better and healthier lifestyle. One that you will feel great about.

The real wisdom and knowledge comes from Dr. Morse, and I encourage each and everyone of you to seek out his website and YouTube videos.
I will put links to those sites in this book below, but if for whatever reason YouTube removes his channel or video's or the address of his website changes, please do yourself a favour and seek him out, everything you could ever need to know will come from him or his associates… that just made me think of another important thing… I told you there is so much to learn about.
I will very briefly tell you that there is a diagnostic tool your body has, and you don't need to go through an x-ray machine or any painful and invasive tests… your eyes. Your eyes can tell you a lot about what is going on inside your body.

It's called Iridology, and Dr. Morse and his trained staff know how to look at your eyes and tell what is currently wrong, what could go wrong, and what can be done to heal you, all from looking at your eyes.

Amazing isn't it!

I will not go any further about Iridology, and please ask you to look for information or videos from Dr. Morse about that.

So, thank you very much for hanging in there and letting me rant and rave about a subject I am pretty passionate about.
I hope that I have opened your eyes and your mind a little more about what is going on with you, and with the world.
If I have helped you in anyway than I am very grateful and happy that my experience and knowledge that I have accumulated on this has been of service.

As promised, here are the links to Dr. Morse's information on the WWW:
Website:
https://www.drmorsesherbalhealthclub.com/

YouTube Channel:
https://www.youtube.com/user/robertmorsend/featured

Thank you and I wish you the very best on your journey.

www.ingramcontent.com/pod-product-compliance
Lightning Source LLC
Chambersburg PA
CBHW031432250726
48656CB00002B/947